Copyright 2023

Table of Contents

Neuropathy is a disorder of the nerves -- the body's system for transmitting messages from the body to the spinal cord and brain, and vice versa. Common symptoms include tingling, numbness, weakness, changes in sensation, and pain.

Neuropathy is a form of nerve damage that is estimated to affect more than 20 million Americans. It often accompanies other health problems including diabetes, cancer, shingles, autoimmune disease or injury.

"Neuropathy presents a spectrum of symptoms," says Daniel DiCapua, MD, a Yale Medicine neurologist. Those symptoms may include a burning sensation, shooting pain, numbness or muscle weakness. For some patients, Dr. DiCapua says, the symptoms are just an annoyance. But for others, the effects of neuropathy can be debilitating.

The team at Yale Medicine has both the comprehensive expertise and advanced equipment to diagnose neuropathy successfully. They also provide treatments that both minimize the discomfort and offer the best opportunity to reverse the condition.

Patients with neuropathy experience "misfiring" of the peripheral nerve cells (nerves that carry signals between the brain and other parts of the body). The result can range from pain to complete loss of sensation.

Up to half of patients with diabetes experience some kind of neuropathic pain.

Other health problems associated with neuropathy include shingles, cancer, autoimmune disease, and certain kind's of injury. It is not clear to researchers exactly why nerve damage results from those conditions.

Early signs of neuropathy can include muscle weakness, twitching or cramps, as well as feelings of numbness or loss of sensation, or lightheadedness.

As the condition progresses, patients might also experience imbalance, emotional distress or trouble sleeping.

Some patients complain of losing sensation in their feet or have problems with motor control. Others feel neuropathic pain in their feet, plus legs, back and hands, which can make the simple act of sitting at a desk—or lying in bed—very difficult.

BREAKFAST

1. Hashbrown Casserole

Prep Time: 20 Minutes

Cook Time: 1hr 10 Minutes

Servings: 8

Ingredients

- 20 ounces shredded hash browns thawed
- 1 pound sausage cooked, crumbled, and drained
- ¼ cup onion finely diced
- ½ red bell pepper diced
- ½ green bell pepper diced
- 2 cups cheddar cheese shredded, divided use
- 8 eggs
- 1 can evaporated milk 12 ounces, or 1 ⅓ cups milk
- ½ teaspoon Italian seasoning or your favorite herbs/spices (optional)
- ½ teaspoon Kosher salt or to taste
- ¼ teaspoon black pepper

Instructions

1. Preheat the oven to 350°F (if baking immediately). Grease a 9×13 inch pan or a 3qt baking dish or spray with cooking spray.

2. Heat a large skillet over medium high heat. Brown the sausage, breaking it up with a spoon, until no pink remains. Drain fat.

3. In the prepared dish, add the hashbrowns, cooked sausage, onions, bell peppers, and 1 ½ cups of cheese. Gently mix the ingredients together and spread evenly in the pan.

4. In a large bowl, add the eggs, evaporated milk, salt & pepper, and Italian seasoning to a large bowl. Whisk until well combined.

5. Pour the egg mixture over the hashbrown mixture and sprinkle the remaining cheese over top.

6. Cover the dish with foil and refrigerate overnight if desired, or bake immediatcly.

7. Bake uncovered for 55-65 minutes or until cooked through.

Prep Time: 20 Minutes

Cook Time: 6hrs 3 Minutes

Servings: 8

Ingredients

- 1 bag frozen hash brown potatoes 32 ounces
- 1 pound bacon, sausage, or ham cooked & cumbled or diced
- 2 cups sharp cheddar cheese shredded, about 8 oz
- 2 green onions sliced
- 1 small finely diced white onion about ½ cup
- 1 red bell pepper diced
- 1 green bell pepper diced
- 12 eggs
- 1 cup milk
- 1 ½ teaspoons dry mustard powder
- 1 teaspoon salt
- 1 teaspoon garlic powder
- ½ teaspoon black pepper

Instructions

1. If using bacon or sausage, cook and crumble. Drain fat leaving 1 tablespoon in the pan.

2. If desired, soften the onion in the fat. This is optional but will soften the flavor of the onion.

3. Grease a 6qt slow cooker. Place half the hash browns, meat, onions, peppers, and cheese in the slow cooker. Repeat layers ending with cheese, do not stir.

4. Whisk eggs, milk, and and seasonings in a medium bowl. Pour the egg mixture over the ingredients in the slow cooker.

5. Cook on low for 7 to 8 hours or high for 3-4 hours. Once cooked, uncover and let the casserole rest for 15 minutes.

Prep Time: 15 Minutes

Cook Time: 60 Minutes

Servings: 8

Ingredients

- 2 teaspoons olive oil
- 1 onion chopped
- 1 clove garlic minced
- ½ red bell pepper finely diced
- ½ green bell pepper finely diced
- 2 cups ham diced
- 8 tortillas 8" each
- 2 cups cheddar cheese shredded, divided
- Egg Mixture
- 5 eggs
- 2 cups milk
- 1 tablespoon flour
- ½ teaspoon oregano
- 3-4 dashes hot sauce such as Tobasco
- Salt & pepper to taste

Instructions

1. Grease a 9x13 baking dish.

2. In a large saucepan, cook onion, garlic and bell peppers in oil over medium heat until tender, about 5 minutes. Stir in ham.

3. Place ¼ cup of ham mixture and 3 tablespoons of cheese on the end of a tortilla. Roll up and place seam side down in prepared pan. Repeat with remaining tortillas.

4. Whisk eggs, milk, flour, oregano, hot sauce, salt and pepper to taste. Pour over tortillas. Cover with foil and refrigerate overnight.

5. Preheat oven to 350°F. Remove pan from fridge while the oven preheats, about 20 minutes.

6. Bake covered for 35 minutes. Remove foil and top with remaining cheese. Bake an additional 15-20 minutes or until eggs are set. Serve with sour cream, salsa and toppings as desired.

Prep Time: 15 Minutes

Cook Time: 10 Minutes

Servings: 4

Ingredients

- 8 eggs
- 1 tablespoon milk
- 1 tablespoon butter
- ¼ cup bell pepper finely diced
- 2 green onions sliced, whites and greens divided
- 1 cup sharp cheddar cheese shredded
- 6 slices bacon cooked and crumbled
- 8 small corn or flour tortillas warmed
- ¼ cup sour cream
- ¼ cup salsa

Instructions

1. In a medium bowl, whisk eggs and milk with salt and pepper to taste.

2. Heat tortillas according to package directions. Wrap in foil to keep warm.

3. In a medium non-stick skillet, melt butter over medium heat. Add the whites of the green onions and the bell peppers. Cook until tender, about 3 minutes.

4. Pour in the egg mixture and scramble gently until set but still shiny.

5. Divide eggs over tortillas. Sprinkle cheese over top and cover for 1 minute to allow the cheese to melt (or broil in the oven for 1 minute if desired).

6. Top with the tops of the green onions and your favorite toppings like crumbled bacon.

7. Serve immediately.

Prep Time: 15 Minutes

Cook Time: 10 Minutes

Servings: 6

Ingredients

- 2 cups all-purpose flour
- 1 tablespoon baking powder
- ½ teaspoon salt
- 2 tablespoons sugar
- 2 large eggs divided
- 1 ⅔ cups milk
- ⅓ Cup melted butter or oil
- 1 teaspoon vanilla extract

Instructions

1. Preheat the waffle iron according to the manufacturer's directions (or to 400°F if your waffle maker has a temperature gauge).
2. Place flour, baking powder, sugar, and salt in a large bowl. Whisk to combine.

3. In a small bowl, mix egg yolks, milk, butter, and vanilla extract. Set aside.

4. In a separate medium bowl, beat egg whites with a mixer on medium high speed until stiff peaks form.

5. Add the egg yolk mixture to the dry ingredients and stir to combine. Gently fold in the egg whites.

6. Drop by large spoonfuls onto greased waffle iron until most of the wells are covered. Close the lid and cook for about 3-5 minutes or until golden brown.

Prep Time: 15 Minutes

Cook Time: 25 Minutes

Servings: 8

Ingredients

- 1 can prepared pizza crust or homemade pizza dough
- 2 tablespoons olive oil
- 6 eggs
- 3 tablespoons milk
- ½ teaspoon dried basil
- Salt & pepper to taste
- ½ pound sausage cooked and drained
- ¼ cup cooked bacon or bacon bits
- 3 green onions sliced, divided
- ¼ cup red bell pepper finely chopped
- 8 ounces Cabot Pepper Jack Cheese
- 2 ounces Cabot Extra Sharp Cheddar

Instructions

1. Preheat oven to 425°F.

2. With 1 tablespoon olive oil, grease a 10"x15" pan with a rim. Press dough into the pan and brush with remaining 1 tablespoon olive oil and sprinkle with basil. Bake 7-8 minutes or until lightly browned.

3. Meanwhile, whisk eggs, milk, and salt & pepper. Cook in a lightly oiled skillet over medium heat just until set, about 3-4 minutes. Eggs should be shiny and undercooked (they will cook more in the oven).

4. Sprinkle pizza with toppings and eggs Sprinkle cheese on top. Bake an additional 8-10 minutes or until cheese is melted.

5. Optional: Broil the pizza for 1-2 minutes to brown the cheese on top.

6. Remove from the oven, sprinkle with parsley. Rest 2-3 minutes before serving.

Prep Time: 20 Minutes

Cook Time: 60 Minutes

Servings: 8

Ingredients

- 12 slices cinnamon bread cut into 1-inch cubes, about 12 cups
- 1 cup carrots shredded
- ⅔ Cup crushed pineapple drained and squeezed very dry
- ½ cup raisins
- 8 eggs
- 2 cups milk
- ⅓ Cup brown sugar
- 1 teaspoon cinnamon
- Cream Cheese Mixture
- 8 ounces cream cheese room temperature
- ¼ cup sugar
- 1 teaspoon orange zest
- Topping
- ¼ cup chopped pecans

- 2 tablespoons butter
- 2 tablespoons flour
- 2 tablespoons flaked coconut
- 1 tablespoon brown sugar
- ½ teaspoon cinnamon

Instructions

1. Leave your bread out for a few hours or place it on a tray at 350°F for about 8 minutes to slightly dry it out.
2. In a medium bowl, combine cream cheese mixture ingredients until fluffy.
3. Grease a 9x13 inch baking dish. Layer half of the bread cubes in the pan. Sprinkle with half of the carrots, pineapple and raisins. Dot with the cream cheese mixture. Top with remaining bread and the other half of the carrots, pineapple, and raisins.
4. In a bowl, stir together the eggs, milk, brown sugar, and cinnamon. Pour over the casserole, cover with foil and refrigerate overnight.
5. Remove the casserole from the fridge about 45-60 minutes before baking. Preheat the oven to 350°F.
6. Mix topping ingredients together in a small bowl. Sprinkle over casserole just before baking.

7. Bake uncovered 45-55 minutes or until a knife inserted
    in the center comes out clean and casserole is set.
8. Cool 15 minutes before serving.

Prep Time: 10 Minutes

Cook Time: 20 Minutes

Servings: 4

Ingredients

- 2 tablespoons olive oil
- ½ cup onion diced
- 4 cups frozen hash browns thawed
- 1 ½ cups leftover ham diced
- ½ green pepper finely diced
- 4 eggs
- Salt and pepper to taste
- ¼ cup cheddar cheese shredded

Instructions

1. Preheat oven to 375°F.
2. Heat olive oil in an ovenproof skillet over medium heat. Add onion and cook until softened, about 5 minutes.

3. Stir in hash browns, ham, and and green peppers. Cook until the hashbrowns are lightly browned, stirring occasionally.

4. Press the back of a spoon into the hashbrowns to create 4 wells. Crack a fresh egg into each well. Season with salt and pepper and top with cheese.

5. Bake for 12-15 minutes or until the eggs are cooked to your preference. The eggs will continue to cook once removed from the oven so do not overcook.

Prep Time: 15 Minutes

Cook Time: 30 Minutes

Servings: 8

Ingredients

- 1 pound breakfast sausage spicy or mild
- 3 cups hash brown potatoes frozen, diced
- 2 tablespoons bell peppers chopped, optional
- 10 large eggs
- ¼ cup milk
- Salt & black pepper to taste
- 1 cup fresh salsa Pico de Gallo is best
- 2 cups sharp cheddar cheese shredded
- 8 12" flour tortillas

Instructions

1. Heat a 12" skillet over medium-high heat and add breakfast sausage, crumbling while cooking. Once browned, spoon onto a paper towel-lined plate leaving about 2 tablespoons of fat in the pan.

2. Add frozen hash browns (and bell peppers if using) to the pan and cook for about 10 minutes or until fully cooked and lightly browned.

3. In a small bowl combine eggs, milk and salt & black to taste. Whisk until fully combined.

4. Remove hash browns from the pan and set aside. Add 1 teaspoon of oil to the pan if needed and reduce heat to medium low.

5. Add eggs and cook until just about set, they will continue cooking as they cool.

6. Arrange 8 pieces of foil with a flour tortilla in the center of each. Divide hash brown mixture, eggs, cheese and salsa over tortillas.

7. Enjoy immediately or wrap the burritos in the foil and store it in a plastic zip-top bag in the freezer.

8. To Reheat

9. Defrost burritos in the fridge overnight for best results. To reheat add to a plate, cover with a paper towel and reheat for about 3 minutes if defrosted or 4 minutes from frozen. Be sure to flip the burrito half way through.

Prep Time: 20 Minutes

Cook Time: 60 Minutes

Servings: 6

Ingredients

- ½ pound sausage
- ½ cup red or green peppers diced
- 6 cups bread cubes slightly dried
- 2 cups cheddar cheese shredded, divided
- Egg Mixture
- 4 eggs
- 1 ½ cups milk
- ½ cup light cream or half and half
- ½ teaspoon dry mustard powder
- ½ teaspoon salt
- ¼ teaspoon pepper
- ¼ teaspoon onion powder

Instructions

1. Cook sausage in a skillet over medium heat until no pink remains, drain the fat and return the sausage to the pan. Add the peppers and cook until slightly tender, about 3 minutes. Set aside to cool.
2. Whisk eggs, milk, cream, dry mustard, salt, pepper, and onion powder in a large bowl (add ½ teaspoon black pepper if desired).
3. Add the bread, peppers, sausage, and half of the cheese to the egg mixture. Toss to combine and let rest for 5 minutes. Toss again until the liquid is absorbed.
4. Add the mixture to a greased 2 qt baking dish. Cover with foil and refrigerate for at least 30 minutes or up to 48 hours.
5. Preheat the oven to 350°F. Bake covered for 30 minutes. Uncover, top with remaining cheese, and bake an additional 15-20 minutes or until set in the middle.
6. Rest 10 minutes before cutting.

11. Homemade Sausages

Prep Time: 10 Minutes

Cook Time: 10 Minutes

Servings: 6

Ingredients

- 1 pound ground pork
- Seasoning Mixture
- 1 teaspoon salt
- ½ teaspoon black pepper
- ½ teaspoon fennel seeds crushed
- ½ teaspoon dried ground sage
- ½ teaspoon garlic powder
- ¼ teaspoon poultry seasoning
- ⅛ Teaspoon thyme leaves
- ⅛ Teaspoon rosemary crushed
- ⅛ Teaspoon smoked paprika
- ⅛ Teaspoon red pepper flakes optional

Instructions

1. Combine pork and all seasonings in a medium bowl. Mix very well.
2. Refrigerate at least 2 hours or overnight.
3. Divide meat into 6 patties, ½" thick.

To Cook

1. Heat a skillet over medium heat.
2. Add patties (and a pat of butter if you'd like) and cook 4 minutes per side or until lightly browned.

Prep Time: 45 Minutes

Cook Time: 15 Minutes

Servings: 6

Ingredients

- 2 pounds Yukon gold potatoes ½ inch pieces
- 1 pound chorizo sausage casing removed
- 4 strips bacon sliced
- 1 onion diced
- 4 cloves garlic minced
- 1 teaspoon coriander
- 1 teaspoon cumin
- ¾ teaspoon smoked paprika
- 6 eggs whisked
- 1 cup cheddar cheese shredded

Instructions

1. Preheat the oven to 375°F.

2. Place the potatoes in a large pot with 6 cups of water, bring to a boil and cook for 6-8 minutes or until they are fork tender. Drain them and set aside.

3. While potatoes are cooking, heat a large skillet over medium heat. Cook the bacon until crisp. Remove and set aside.

4. Remove the casing from the chorizo and add it to the bacon fat along with the onion. Cook until no pink remains, about 8 minutes. Remove from the pan and set aside leaving the fat in the pan.

5. Turn the heat up to medium high and add the potatoes, seasonings, and and garlic to the pan. Cook until browned without stirring too much so the potatoes can form a crust. Stir in the meat.

6. While potatoes are browning, lightly scramble the eggs in a small pan over medium heat. Eggs should be slightly undercooked and shiny. Place on top of the hash and sprinkle cheese on top.

7. Place in the oven and heat until cheese is melted and heat through, about 5 minutes.

Prep Time: 10 Minutes

Cook Time: 20 Minutes

Servings: 12

Ingredients

- 12 Hawaiian rolls or dinner rolls or slider buns
- 12 slices deli ham
- 8 ounces sliced Swiss cheese or cheddar cheese
- 6 tablespoons butter melted, divided
- 1 ½ teaspoons Dijon mustard or grainy mustard
- 1 teaspoon Worcestershire sauce
- 1 teaspoon poppy seeds
- 1 teaspoon dried minced onion

Instructions

1. Preheat the oven to 350°F.
2. In a small bowl combine 4 tablespoons melted butter, Dijon mustard, Worcestershire sauce, poppy seeds, and dried minced onion.

3. Cut the rolls in half separating the top and bottom. If they are attached you don't need to separate each roll.

4. Brush with the inside of the rolls remaining 2 tablespoons butter.

5. Place the bottom of the rolls in a baking dish. Layer a slice of folded ham on each roll and top with cheese slices.

6. Place the top half of the rolls on the cheese and gently brush the butter mixture over top.

7. Bake uncovered for about 20 minutes or until the cheese has melted and the tops are lightly browned.

8. Serve warm and enjoy.

Prep Time: 20 Minutes

Cook Time: 10 Minutes

Servings: 6

Ingredients

- 1 ½ pounds fresh Brussels sprouts shredded
- 1 medium apple granny smith, or any variety
- 1 teaspoon lemon juice
- ⅓ Cup dried cranberries or dried cherries
- ⅓ Cup pomegranate arils
- ¼ cup walnuts or pecans, chopped
- 2 ounces feta cheese crumbled
- Dressing
- ⅓ Cup olive oil
- 3 tablespoons cider vinegar
- 2 tablespoons honey
- 1 tablespoon fresh lemon juice
- 1 ½ teaspoons dijon mustard
- ½ teaspoon garlic powder
- Salt and pepper to tastes

Instructions

1. In a small jar, combine olive oil, cider vinegar, honey, lemon juice, Dijon mustard, garlic powder, salt, and pepper. Shake well to mix.
2. Toast the nuts in a dry skillet over medium heat, stirring frequently, until they are fragrant and lightly browned, about 4 minutes.
3. Shred Brussels sprouts, rinse well, and dry.
4. Chop the apple and toss with 1 teaspoon lemon juice.
5. In a large salad bowl, combine Brussels sprouts, apple, dried cranberries, pomegranate arils, walnuts, and feta cheese.
6. Drizzle with dressing, toss to coat, and serve.

Prep Time: 15 Minutes

Cook Time: 25 Minutes

Servings: 4

Ingredients

- 4 chicken breast halves skinless boneless
- ½ cup all-purpose flour
- 2 large eggs
- ⅔ Cup Panko bread crumbs
- ⅔ Cup Italian seasoning bread crumbs
- ⅓ Cup parmesan cheese grated
- 2 tablespoons fresh parsley
- 4 tablespoons olive oil or as needed
- 24 ounces marinara sauce homemade or jarred
- 1 cup mozzarella cheese shredded
- ¼ cup Parmesan cheese shredded
- 1 teaspoon basil fresh, chopped, for garnish
- 1 teaspoon parsley fresh, chopped, for garnish

Instructions

1. Preheat the oven to 425°F.

2. Place the flour in a shallow bowl or dish. Place the eggs in a second shallow dish and beat with a fork.

3. In a third shallow dish, combine Panko, Italian seasoned crumbs, grated Parmesan, 2 tablespoons fresh parsley, ½ teaspoon salt, and ¼ teaspoon pepper.

4. Using a meat mallet, pound the chicken breasts to ½-inch thickness. After pounding, if they're very large, you can cut them in half. Pat the chicken dry with paper towels and season with ½ teaspoon salt and ¼ teaspoon black pepper.

5. Dip chicken into the flour and shake to remove any excess. Dip chicken in beaten eggs, then into the bread crumb mixture and gently press to adhere.

6. Preheat the oil over medium-high heat in a large skillet. Brown the chicken for about 2 minutes per side or until golden. It does not need to cook through.

7. In the bottom of a 9×13 baking dish, add 1 ½ cups of marinara sauce. Add the browned chicken. Top each piece of chicken with 2 tablespoons of marinara sauce in the center. Top with mozzarella and shredded parmesan.

8. Bake for 20-25 minutes or until golden and bubbly and the chicken reaches an internal temperature of 165°F with an instant-read thermometer.

9. Sprinkle with fresh herbs and serve over pasta.

Prep Time: 10 Minutes

Cook Time: 10 Minutes

Servings: 4

Ingredients

- 8 eggs hard boiled and cooled
- ½ cup mayonnaise
- 1 ½ teaspoons yellow mustard
- 1 green onion thinly sliced
- 1 rib celery finely diced
- 2 teaspoons fresh dill chopped

Instructions

1. Cut eggs in half. Remove yolks and chop whites.
2. Mash yolks with mayonnaise, mustard and salt & pepper to taste until smooth and creamy.
3. Add remaining ingredients and stir well.
4. Serve on bread or over lettuce.

Prep Time: 15 Minutes

Cook Time: 18 Minutes

Servings: 6

Ingredients

- 3 cups egg noodles
- 1 tablespoon butter
- 1 small onion diced
- 2 stalks celery diced
- ⅔ Cup frozen peas defrosted
- 1 can tuna 5-6 ounces, drained
- 10 ½ ounces condensed cream of mushroom soup
- ⅓ Cup milk
- 1 cup cheddar cheese
- 1 tablespoon parsley
- Crumb Topping
- ½ cup panko bread crumbs
- 1 tablespoon butter melted
- ½ cup cheddar
- 1 tablespoon parsley

Instructions

1. Preheat oven to 425°F. Combine topping ingredients and set aside.
2. Boil noodles al dente according to package directions. Drain and rinse under cold water.
3. Cook onion and celery in butter until tender, about 5-7 minutes.
4. In a large bowl combine noodles, onion mixture, peas, soup, milk, cheese, tuna and parsley. Mix well.
5. Spread into a 2qt casserole dish and top with crumb topping.
6. Bake 18-20 minutes or until bubbly.

Prep Time: 20 Minutes

Cook Time: 1hr 20 Minutes

Servings: 60

Ingredients

Dough

- 6 cups all-purpose flour
- 2 cups cold water divided
- 2 eggs beaten
- 6 tablespoons canola or vegetable oil
- 2 teaspoons salt

Filling

- 3 ¾ pounds baking potatoes
- 1 medium white onion finely diced
- ⅓ Cup softened butter divided
- 4 ½ cups cheddar cheese finely shredded
- Salt to taste
- White pepper to taste, or very fine black pepper

For Serving

- 1 onion diced or thinly sliced
- 2 tablespoons butter or as needed for frying
- Sour cream optional, for serving

Instructions

Dough

1. In a large bowl add flour, eggs, oil, salt, and 1 ½ cups of water. Mix well to form a dough, adding more water if needed.
2. Knead the dough on a flat surface for about 4 to 5 minutes or until it becomes smooth and pliable.
3. Cover the dough with plastic wrap and let it rest at room temperature for at least 30 minutes or up to 1 hour.

Filling

1. Peel the potatoes and cut them into 2-inch cubes. Place them in a large pot of salted water and bring to a boil. Cook the potatoes for 15 minutes or until fork tender.
2. While the potatoes are cooking, in a medium skillet over medium-low heat, cook the onions in 2 tablespoons butter until tender without browning.

3. Once the potatoes are cooked, place them in a large bowl and mash them. Add onions, cheese, and remaining butter. Continue mashing until the potatoes become very smooth.

Assembly

1. Using half of the dough, roll it out ⅛" thick. Cut out circles of dough using a 3" cookie or biscuit cutter.
2. Scoop 1 ½ tablespoons of filling and roll into a ball, place on the pierogi dough. Fold the dough over to form a semi-circle and pinch the edges closed. Place on a baking sheet. Repeat.
3. The pierogi can either be cooked or frozen at this point.

To Cook

1. Heat 3 tablespoons butter in a large skillet. Add diced onions and cook on medium-low heat until tender. Remove onions from the pan and set aside for serving.
2. Bring a large pot of salted water to a boil. Gently add pierogies and cook until they float, about 2 to 4 minutes. Remove with a slotted spoon.
3. Transfer pierogies to the hot skillet (adding more butter if needed) and cook until browned on each side, about 5 minutes.
4. Serve warm with onions and sour cream.

Prep Time: 10 Minutes

Cook Time: 15 Minutes

Servings: 2

Ingredients

- 1 tomato sliced
- 2 english muffins halved
- 2 ounces cheddar cheese
- Tuna Salad
- 6 ounces white flaked tuna in water drained
- 1 stalk celery finely diced
- 1 green onion sliced
- ⅓ Cup mayonnaise
- 1 teaspoon dijon
- ½ teaspoon lemon juice
- Salt & pepper to taste

Instructions

1. Preheat oven to 400°F.

2. Combine tuna salad ingredients in a small bowl and mix well.

3. Place the English muffin halves on a baking sheet and broil 2-3 minutes or until they start to brown. Remove from the oven.

4. Divide the tuna mixture over the English muffins. Top with tomato slices and cheddar cheese.

5. Bake 10-15 minutes or until cheese is melted. Broil 1 minute if desired.

20. Classic Grilled Cheese Sandwich

Prep Time: 5 Minutes

Cook Time: 7 Minutes

Servings: 2

Ingredients

- 4 slices white bread or sour dough
- 2 tablespoons mayonnaise
- 4 ounces cheddar cheese or American cheese
- 2 tablespoons shredded cheddar optional

Instructions

1. Preheat a small skillet over low heat.
2. Spread mayonnaise over one side of each piece of bread and place mayonnaise side down in the skillet.
3. Top with cheddar cheese slices, black pepper to taste and remaining slice of bread, mayonnaise side out.
4. Grill until golden, about 4-5 minutes. Flip and grill the other side until golden.

5. Optional: Just before serving, add the shredded cheddar directly to the outside of the sandwich and grill an additional minute or so until it gets crispy.

21. Cheesy Stuffed Biscuits

Prep Time: 10 Minutes

Cook Time: 10 Minutes

Servings: 10

Ingredients

- 3 ounces deli ham diced
- ½ cup cheddar cheese shredded
- 1 tablespoon butter melted
- ½ teaspoon Dijon optional
- 1 can refrigerated biscuits 16 ounces
- 1 teaspoon sesame seeds

Instructions

1. Preheat oven to 375°F. Grease a muffin tin.
2. In a small bowl, combine diced ham and cheese. In a separate small bowl, mix together melted butter and Dijon if using.
3. Gently cut biscuit open, like a sandwich bun, stopping ¼-inch from the end.

4. Open the biscuit and place 1 tablespoon of ham and cheese mixture in the middle of the dough.

5. Close the biscuit and seal the edges by pinching all the way around. Repeat with remaining biscuits.

6. Place biscuits in the muffin pan. Brush with the Dijion/butter mixture, and sprinkle with sesame seeds.

7. Bake for 10 to 12 minutes or browned. Do not over bake.

8. Cool in pan for 5 minutes.

Prep Time: 5 Minutes

Cook Time: 7 Minutes

Servings: 8

- Ingredients
- 8 slices bread crusts removed
- 8 slices cheese or more to taste, or 1 cup+ grated cheddar
- 8 slices bacon raw or pre-cooked
- ¼ cup butter

Instructions

1. If using raw bacon, partially cook it in the air fryer or in a frying pan over medium high heat until some of the fat has rendered out. Ensure the bacon is not cooked too crispy.
2. Cut the crusts off of the bread if desired. Use a rolling pin to roll the bread flat.
3. Place one slice of cheese (or more if you'd like) or 2-3 tablespoons shredded cheese on each slice.

4. Roll up the bread and cheese. Wrap one slice of bacon around each roll and secure with a toothpick on each end.

5. Place in a pan over medium-low heat. Add a small spoonful of butter & using tongs, rub the rolls in the butter ensuring the bread edges are covered.

6. Continue adding bits of butter and turning with tongs until all sides are browned and cheese is melted.

7. Serve immediately.

Prep Time: 10 Minutes

Cook Time: 10 Minutes

Servings: 4

Ingredients

- 1 small onion diced
- 2 stalks celery
- 2 tablespoons butter
- 8 cups fresh cauliflower
- 3 cups chicken broth
- ½ teaspoon celery seed
- ½ teaspoon dry mustard powder
- ½ teaspoon garlic powder
- ¼ teaspoon seasoning salt
- ¾ cup heavy cream
- ½ cup fresh parmesan cheese grated, optional

Instructions

1. Heat butter in a medium saucepan over medium heat. Cook onion and celery until tender (do not brown).

2. Add cauliflower, broth and seasonings. Simmer uncovered 10-15 minutes stirring occasionally until cauliflower is tender.

3. Blend using a hand blender until smooth. Add heavy cream and simmer an additional 8-10 minutes or until thickened.

4. Season with salt & pepper to taste. Stir in parmesan cheese if using.

24. One Pan Turkey

Prep Time: 30 Minutes

Cook Time: 1hr 25 Minutes

Servings: 4

Ingredients

Stuffing

- ½ cup onion finely diced
- ½ cup celery finely diced
- ⅓ Cup butter
- ¾ teaspoon poultry seasoning
- 6 cups stale/dry bread cubes about 8 slices of bread
- 1 tablespoon fresh herbs I used parsley, thyme, and sage
- 1 ½ to 2 cups chicken broth
- Salt & pepper to taste

Turkey

- 2 pounds boneless turkey breast with skin
- 2 teaspoons olive oil
- ¼ teaspoon poultry seasoning

- 1 tablespoon fresh herbs I used parsley, thyme, and sage
- Salt & pepper

Potatoes

- 1 ½ pounds yellow potatoes
- ½ onion thinly sliced
- 1 teaspoon fresh rosemary finely minced
- ½ teaspoon garlic powder
- ½ cup heavy cream
- Pats of butter to taste
- Cranberry Sauce
- 1 ½ cups cranberries about 6 ounces
- ½ cup sugar
- Pinch cinnamon
- 1 tablespoon orange juice or water
- Brussels sprouts
- 1 pound brussels sprouts
- 2 slices bacon uncooked, chopped
- 1 teaspoon olive oil

Instructions

Pan

1. Preheat oven to 375°F.

2. Line a large 18"x13" sheet pan with Reynolds Wrap®
    Heavy Duty Foil. Divide the tray into sections using
    foil. The first section is for the turkey and stuffing,
    about 8" of the pan. Make the middle section about 5"
    for the potatoes and the last section will be 5" for the
    brussels sprouts. Generously spray each section with
    cooking spray (or use Reynolds Wrap® Non-Stick Foil
    to keep food from sticking). Set aside.

Stuffing

1. Cook onion & celery in butter with poultry seasoning
    over medium-low heat until tender but not browned,
    about 10 minutes.

2. Combine bread cubes, onion mixture & herbs in a bowl.
    Toss with broth, a little bit at a time until bread is moist
    (but not soggy). You may not need all of the broth.
    Season with salt and pepper to taste. Set aside.

Turkey

1. Rub the outside of the turkey breast with oil. Sprinkle
    with poultry seasoning and fresh herbs and season

generously with salt & pepper. Place in the largest section of the pan. Arrange stuffing around the turkey breast and place pats of butter on the stuffing if desired.

Potatoes

2. Bring a large pot of water to a boil.

3. Scrub the potatoes and slice ¼″ thick. Boil 5 minutes or just until tender-crisp. During the last minute of cooking, add the sliced onions to the water. Drain well.

4. Toss the potatoes with rosemary, garlic powder, and salt & pepper. Place in the middle section of the pan. Drizzle with the cream and add pats of butter on top of the potatoes.

Cranberry Sauce

1. Combine sauce ingredients and place in 1 or two small oven-proof bowls (this will need to expand so allow extra space in the bowl). Cover with foil and nestle the bowls in the sections where you have space.

Brussels sprouts

2. Rinse brussels sprouts and drain well. Remove any discolored leaves and cut in half if large. Toss with oil

and season with salt & pepper. Set aside (these will be added later in cooking).

Baking

3. Place the sheet pan in the middle of the oven and bake 25 minutes. Add brussels sprouts and uncooked bacon to the remaining section. Bake an additional 25-35 minutes or until turkey is cooked to 165°F.
4. Remove from the oven and rest 15 minutes before serving.
5. While the turkey is resting, remove the foil from the cranberry sauce, stir and transfer to a cool bowl.
6. Toss Brussels and bacon to combine. Slice the turkey breast and serve.

Prep Time: 20 Minutes

Cook Time: 35 Minutes

Servings: 8

Ingredients

- 6 cups fresh broccoli cut into bite sized pieces
- 2 cups cooked white rice

SAUCE

- 3 tablespoons butter
- ¾ cup onion diced (about 1 small)
- 3 tablespoons flour
- 2 cups milk
- ¼ teaspoon each garlic & black pepper
- ½ teaspoon dry mustard powder
- ½ teaspoon paprika
- Salt to taste
- 3 tablespoons cream cheese
- 2 cups shredded cheddar cheese divided

Instructions

1. Preheat oven to 350°F.

2. Cook onion and butter on medium-low heat until softened and translucent. Stir in flour, garlic powder and pepper. Cook an additional 2 minutes.

3. Gradually pour in milk while whisking. Continue whisking over medium heat until thick and bubbly. Remove from heat and add dry mustard, paprika, cream cheese and 1 ½ cups cheddar cheese. Stir until melted. Taste and season the sauce with salt and pepper.

4. Place broccoli in boiling water for about 2 minutes. You still want it slightly crisp as it cooks more in the oven.

5. Stir together rice, broccoli and cheese sauce. Place in a greased 2 qt casserole dish. Top with remaining cheese and bake 35 minutes or until bubbly and cheese lightly browned.

26. Monterey Chicken

Prep Time: 10 Minutes

Cook Time: 30 Minutes

Servings: 4

Ingredients

- 4 chicken breasts skinless & boneless
- 1 cup bbq sauce
- Salt and pepper to taste
- 1 cup cheese shredded
- ½ cup tomatoes diced
- ¼ cup bacon bits
- 2 green onions sliced

Instructions

1. Preheat the oven to 350°F.
2. Season the chicken with salt and pepper and toss with half of the bbq sauce. Spread the remaining bbq sauce into the bottom of the 9x13 pan or 2.5 qt baking dish.
3. Add the chicken to the dish and cook for 20-25 minutes or until the chicken reaches 165°F in the thickest part.

4. Top with shredded cheese and broil for 1-2 minutes or until melted.

5. Sprinkle with tomatoes*, bacon bits, & green onions, and serve.

Prep Time: 20 Minutes

Cook Time: 3hrs 30 Minutes

Servings: 12

Ingredients

- 1 cup butter
- ½ teaspoon black pepper
- ½ teaspoon salt or to taste
- 2 teaspoons poultry seasoning store bought or homemade
- 2 medium onions diced
- 2 cups celery chopped
- 6 cups cubed and dried white bread
- 6 cups cubed and dried brown bread
- ¼ cup chopped parsley
- 1 tablespoon fresh herbs, or more to taste thyme, sage, rosemary (optional)
- 3-4 cups chicken broth
- 2 eggs

Instructions

1. Heat butter over medium heat until melted. Stir in poultry seasoning, black pepper and salt to taste. Add celery & onions and cook until softened (do not brown). Cool completely.
2. Place bread cubes in a large bowl. Add cooled celery and onion mixture, parsley and fresh herbs if using.
3. Add chicken broth a little bit at a time just to moisten and gently stir. You may not need all of the broth (see note below). Stir in eggs.
4. Cover and refrigerate overnight if making ahead of time.
5. Grease a 5-6 qt slow cooker well. Place stuffing in the slow cooker and turn onto high for 30 minutes. Reduce temperature to low and cook an additional 3-4 hours or until hot and cooked through. If stuffing is done before your meal is ready it can remain on warm.

Prep Time: 10 Minutes

Cook Time: 20 Minutes

Servings: 4

Ingredients

- 4 chicken breasts 7-8 ounces each
- ½ teaspoon chili powder
- Salt & pepper to taste
- 15 ounces black beans drained & rinsed
- 2 cups whole kernel corn
- 1 cup diced bell peppers any color
- ¾ cup salsa or 10 ounces Rotel Diced Tomatoes & Green Chilies, drained
- ½ cup Mexican cheese or monterey jack, shredded
- Cilantro tomatoes & jalapenos for garnish

Instructions

1. Preheat grill to medium-high heat.
2. Place four large pieces of foil on work surface and spray each with cooking spray. Place 1 chicken breast on each

piece of foil and season with chili powder, salt &
pepper.

3. Divide beans, corn, peppers, and salsa over top of
chicken breasts.

4. Fold in the ends to seal each packet. Place packets the
grill vegetable side down for 10 minutes.

5. Flip packets over and grill an additional 10-12 minutes
or until chicken is cooked through and reaches 165°F.

6. Place packets on a large baking pan. Carefully open
packets and top with cheese. Place the baking pan back
on the grill to melt the cheese.

7. Top as desired.

Prep Time: 20 Minutes

Cook Time: 30 Minutes

Servings: 4

Ingredients

- 3 lbs potatoes cut ¼" slices
- 1 small onion thinly
- 3 tablespoons butter
- Salt & pepper to taste

Optional Toppings

- Mushrooms
- Real bacon bits
- Cheese

Instructions

1. Place foil packets on the counter and spray with cooking spray.
2. Wash and slice potatoes (and onions/mushrooms if using).

3. Place potato slices (approx 1 potato per packet) and any optional toppings on each foil piece. Top with a generous pat of butter and salt/pepper to taste. Fold each packet closed.

4. Grill over medium heat for 30 minutes or until soft.

Prep Time: 20 Minutes

Cook Time: 20 Minutes

Servings: 8

Ingredients

- 1 pound jumbo lump crab meat
- ¼ cup mayonnaise
- 1 large egg beaten
- 1 tablespoon Dijon mustard
- 1 tablespoon Worcestershire sauce
- 1 teaspoon Old Bay seasoning
- ½ cup panko bread crumbs unflavored
- 1 ½ tablespoons finely chopped fresh parsley
- 1 teaspoon lemon zest
- ½ teaspoon Kosher salt or to taste
- ½ teaspoon pepper or to taste
- ¼ cup canola oil
- Lemon wedges for serving

Instructions

1. Check the crab meat for any hard and sharp cartilage, remove, and discard.

2. In a bowl, whisk together mayonnaise, beaten egg, Dijon mustard, Worcestershire sauce, and Old Bay seasoning.

3. Add crab meat, bread crumbs, parsley, lemon zest, salt, and pepper. Gently fold to combine, being careful not to break up the crab.

4. Gently press to shape into 6-8 crab cakes using ⅓ cup each, then place on a plate. Cover with plastic wrap and refrigerate for at least 1 hour.

5. Heat the oil in a large nonstick over medium heat. Cook the crab cakes 3-5 minutes per side or until golden brown.

6. Serve immediately with tartar sauce and lemon wedges.